Dear Susan...
'Lord D....'
& the going down of the sun on the NHS...!
(or is there still hope?)

Len Bartholomew (LB)

A third paperback of the Dear Susan... *trilogy*

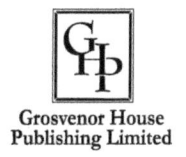

Grosvenor House
Publishing Limited

All rights reserved
Copyright © Len Bartholomew, 2025

The right of Len Bartholomew to be identified as the author of this work has been asserted in accordance with Section 78 of the Copyright, Designs and Patents Act 1988

The book cover is copyright to Len Bartholomew

This book is published by
Grosvenor House Publishing Ltd
Link House
140 The Broadway, Tolworth, Surrey, KT6 7HT.
www.grosvenorhousepublishing.co.uk

This book is sold subject to the conditions that it shall not, by way of trade or otherwise, be lent, resold, hired out or otherwise circulated without the author's or publisher's prior consent in any form of binding or cover other than that in which it is published and without a similar condition including this condition being imposed on the subsequent purchaser.

A CIP record for this book
is available from the British Library

ISBN 978-1-83615-173-9

Front and back covers – the beach and harbour wall, Greece – with the sunshine filtered out.

"Don't judge a book by its cover" – George Eliot

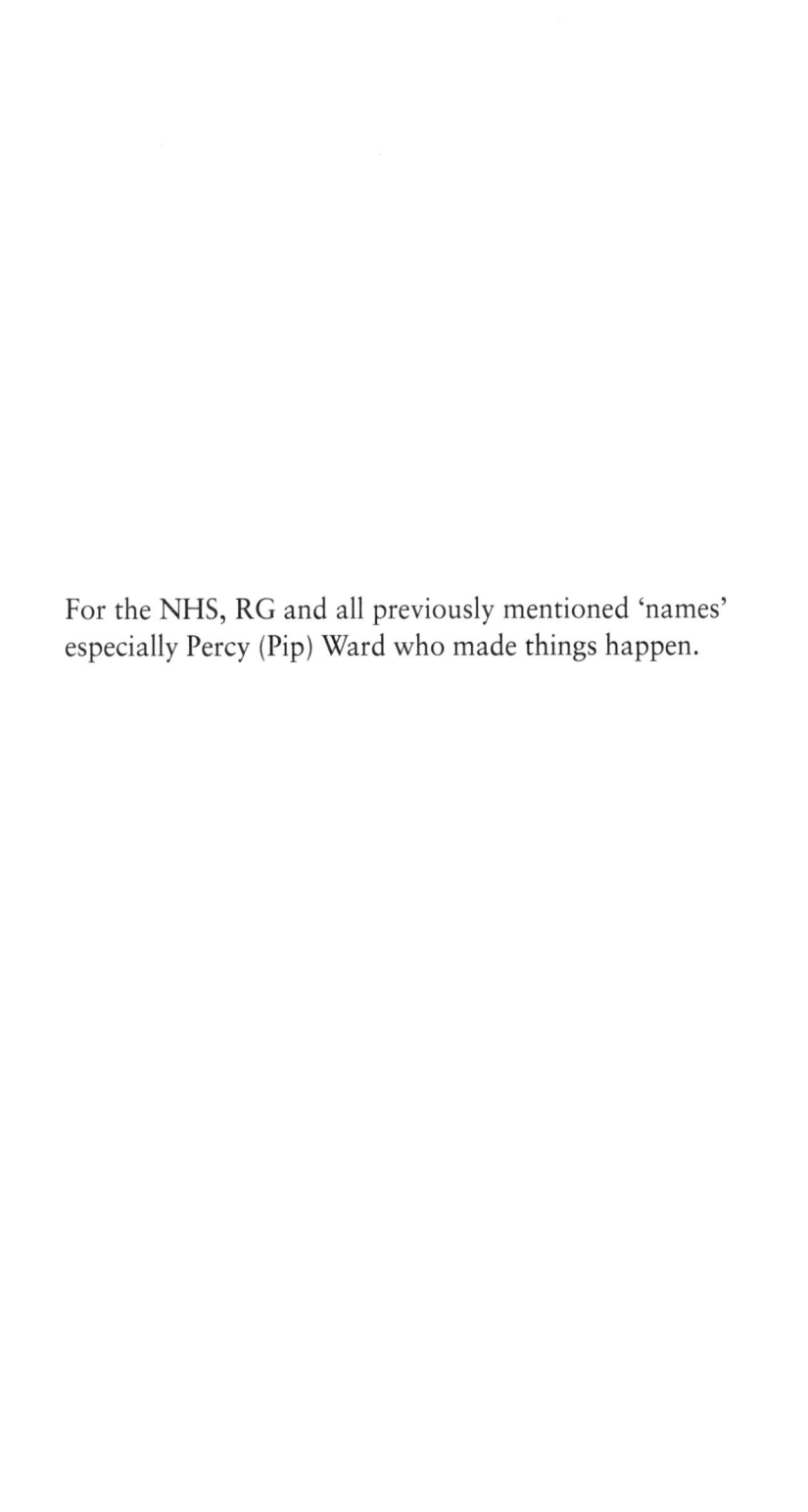

For the NHS, RG and all previously mentioned 'names' especially Percy (Pip) Ward who made things happen.

Dear Susan is the secretary to three orthopaedic surgeons at St George's Hospital. Her contribution is recorded for posterity in the first '*Dear Susan... don't drink and decorate... (a blueprint for the NHS?)*' paperback published on 13th July 2023 with heartfelt thanks.

It is grossly unfair that we have to rely so heavily on the Dear Susans working in the NHS to run many extra miles for patients unable to fend for themselves. A timely and successful healthcare pathway from "sickness to health" or from admission to discharge and beyond through a period of rehabilitation with improved notifications and communications should be the responsibility of all NHS staff no matter what their job description – for all patients.

It makes so much sense to provide staff with the right facilities and equipment to get on with their tasks which are difficult enough without having to work in inferior or failing hospital buildings that straight-jacket the whole process.

Foreword

There really is no way of stopping LB – he will keep going until he drops or requires another dose of the NHS in an out-of-date hospital building!

Even though he knows that hardly anyone is listening or reading his message, it is beyond LB's comprehension that any government would choose to allow the NHS to lurch from crisis to crisis. Lord Darzi confirmed in no uncertain terms* that the NHS needs repairing even if it is not "broken" (official government terminology). Surely someone must want to find a way to fix the NHS estate to help make it fully functional again?

So, if you are a reader, would you mind bearing with LB one more time as he again tries to make the case that by putting the NHS infrastructure in order and in providing smaller hospitals quickly, all other issues might pale into insignificance.

At least his illustrations are pretty if not decipherable and they might help prove he has a point to make to his doubters!

RG

January 2025

---

* Lord Darzi's ("Lord D....") report "Independent Investigation of the NHS in England" 12th September 2024.

Preface

A letter to the editor of the RIBA Journal published in its August 2020 edition:

Horrible hospitals

RE 'Medical mutations' (RIBAJ, p38) I am not sure whether Christopher Shaw is speaking on behalf of Architects for Health or offering a personal view but my own opinion is that, following the first bout of Covid-19, we should avoid building 'European super hospitals' just as we should avoid if possible Covid-19. We should use those many hospital sites he mentions to build smarter, smaller hospitals that people (patients, their visitors and staff) can confidently access when they have to. These should be as unlike the nightmarish Nightingale hospitals as possible.

A large hospital is too big for patients and staff to comprehend and cannot be patient-focussed because its maze of rooms and corridors misinform, disorientate and increase dependency. When it facilitates bad practice, it is not easily changed and because of its size and complexity, almost impossible to replace. Large hospitals have always become obsolete too soon and unmanageable for too long. We have had decades to understand this in project after project.

LB – (former hospital planner and former member of Architects for Health) August 2020

The above letter was written over four years ago. It is b***** outrageous that so little has changed in this time!

My first *Dear Susan...* paperback described, amongst other things, a possible blueprint for the NHS after a recent spell in hospital. Not much interest there then? My second *Dear Susan...* paperback was equally unsuccessful in getting across its message that the NHS estate has fallen into disrepair and needs fixing. Also, that an answer to solving this issue might be to consider constructing smaller hospitals quickly, rather than taking decades to plan larger hospitals via thousands of totally misinformed meetings involving too many key medical staff. This might assist hard-done-by frontline staff to begin to help the NHS to recover for the sake of all patients.

I became convinced that a third Dear Susan... was needed to complete a trilogy of unsuccessful, unread messages to my non-responsive "target audience". I now believe, following Lord Darzi's review, that my paperbacks are more relevant to the government's ten-year plan promised for spring 2025 than my "target audience" was ever likely to understand. Lord Darzi set the cat amongst the pigeons by pointing out the challenges facing the NHS. I think it is now time to deal with the "crumbling" buildings he describes and the state of the NHS and its estate in a planned and comprehensive way.

I hope this third paperback is not cluttered by too many words – other than those that might introduce or explain a series of illustrations as captions.

I have resorted to doing what most architects do when communicating by using diagrams with very few words to avoid architectural jargon that no one understands – especially architects. The idea being that a paperback with a few photos and uncomplicated coloured plans might be left on a dusty shelf to show that in the aftermath of the first wave of the Covid pandemic in 2020, not everyone was struck silent. There were a few ideas floating about which attempted to face up to this crisis.

Since then, it has been decided by a lot of people that nothing should be done about the state of our NHS hospital estate and in not doing so the health of the nation.

To avoid a need for readers to refer back to the previous two issues of the *Dear Susan...* trilogy, the target audience was/is as follows:

- Dear Susan and Mr Consultant – with many thanks
- Chair of St George's, Epsom and St Helier University Hospitals Health Group
- Dear Chief Transformation Officer – St George's Hospital
- Local District and GP Nursing Services
- Dear Clare – South-west London NHS
- Secretary of State for Health and Social Care
- Shadow Secretary of State for Health and Social Care
- Former Chair of the Health and Social Care Committee – 2020-2022

- Former Chair of the Health and Social Care Committee – up to 2024
- Minister of Health – 1975
- Medical Director – NHS England
- Mole Valley District Council
- *A Times* columnist
- The BBC Health Editor and two BBC journalists
- RIBA publications
- Architects for Health
- President of the Royal College of Surgeons – England

In a hope that a few others might prove to be more interested, the following additional names were targeted following the publication of the *Dear Susan…* sequel in May 2024:

- Chief Executive – NHS England
- Chief Executive King's Fund
- CMO East Surrey Hospital – one of the first nucleus hospitals
- The former prime minister!
- The former chancellor of the exchequer!
- The editor of *The Times*
- The editor of the *Architects Journal*
- Various architects

These lists are not about naming names, they are more about showing how even those in positions of power seem to be busy doing little or nothing to sort out the NHS – what is the problem with everyone?

Or, is there a glimmer of hope from the 30th October 2024 Budget funding announcements? The chancellor of the exchequer, when speaking to journalists and the BBC on Monday 28th October about a first but not final word, said, 'The NHS *was the lifeblood of Britain*' and that is why she is '*putting an end to the neglect and the underinvestment it has seen for over a decade. We will be known as the government that took the NHS from its worst crisis in its history, got it back on its feet again and made it fit for the bright future ahead of it.*'

I hope this third paperback of my *Dear Susan...* trilogy can be put to use and that it is not destined to become, like any old retread/historical manuscript, found only in libraries where the odd, odd-ball researcher might find it hidden away for future reference – not so much a legacy, more a waste of time!

LB

January 2025

Contents

Introduction	1
Chapter 1 – Dear Mungo & 10,000m^2 v 90,000m^2 hospitals	7
Chapter 2 – Trauma & Elective Care Centres	15
Chapter 3 – So, what about other specialties?	31
Chapter 4 – May the 4-story limit be exceeded?	35
Chapter 5 – Reasons offered up for doing nothing!	41
Chapter 6 – Smaller Hospitals should be…?	47
Chapter 7 – Next steps?	51
Chapter 8 – A machine for healing?	55
Acknowledgements	61
Appendix	63
A Chorus for all to sing!	65
A final prompt!	67
A photo; 'the going down of the sun'	71

Introduction

Lord Darzi's (Lord D....) review published on 12th September 2024 gave a thumbs down to the state and performance of the NHS over the last decade. It is expected that this review will provide the inspiration for this government's new ten-year plan for the NHS – or will it?

The BBC News summary the following day included the following quotes from this review amongst many other criticisms/observations:

> "The NHS should aspire to deliver high quality care for all, all of the time"

> "We should drive up productivity in hospitals. Acute care providers will need to bring down waiting lists by radically improving their performance. That means fixing flow through by better operational management, capital investment in modern buildings and equipment and re engaging and empowering staff"

LB's blueprint for the NHS in his first Dear Susan... paperback followed on from his time spent as an inpatient in 2020. This focussed on the kind of hospitals he thought were now needed to help restore confidence

INTRODUCTION

in the NHS and to get the nation back on its feet again – after the Covid pandemic[1].

LB had previously found that many existing large hospitals were obsolete. Some were found to be obsolete before they were commissioned because they take too long to plan and build. Given the state of the current batch of hospitals, these are at best only able to prepare patients for the least satisfactory outcomes. They seem hardly ever able to provide timely, consistent, corrective treatment for disabling injuries and illnesses. Nowadays in the UK, most patients are expected to join a huge waiting list. Many patients are likely to have a long wait without treatment, including some patients who wait untreated until they pop off! Large hospitals often give the impression that they favour only dealing with interesting injuries and illnesses that might advance medical knowledge and reputations. Why this should be so when there is a massive backlog of conditions that are known to be treatable begs the question. Large hospitals can be internal, self- interested organisations/institutions with mostly despondent staff who feel undervalued, as do their patients.

Please discuss – is this true[2] and is there an alternative?

---

[1] During the early 1990s, LB, assisted by a large multidisciplinary team of enthusiasts, was asked to review the results of the hospital building programme and the building of nucleus hospitals from 1970-1990 and to update the database. Also, to look forward to make predictions about future provision.

[2] On the 13th November 2024, the secretary of state promised "a no-holds-barred sweeping review" of NHS performance in England.

Yes! It has been staring us in the face for decades, but nothing is new[3]

A return to smaller hospitals located in the community makes sense having tried and tested failing larger hospitals over many decades. New smaller hospitals in many more community locations could provide an opportunity to increase communications, be proactive, responsive and ready to deliver creative outcomes for all age groups from a fully informed clinical regime alert to early diagnosis and a need to take immediate action. They would be in a better position to do their utmost to treat and discharge patients quickly – having put them back on their feet to get back to school, work or to enjoy retirement.

In 2020, Covid came to call to confirm a change was desperately needed – what further proof do we require?

So why not abandon all plans to build large hospital projects? Instead, why not get on quickly with constructing a network of new, easy, fast, smart, smaller hospitals to deal with urgent, newly presented cases and also to tackle the massive backlog of patients on that interminable waiting list?

Patients need procedures for a wide range of surgical and medical conditions. Let us get moving/mobile to recharge batteries to make the UK a healthier place by

---

[3] See also MAAP Architects with Fleet Architects and Durrow Management 2021 Wolfson Economics Prize shortlisted entry – in anticipation of a real and obvious need for change.

INTRODUCTION

building a few smaller hospitals quickly with direct links to all other local health, social care and wellbeing services – for starters.

Oh dear! Let it be, let it be! No! We need efficient healing machines not large, static, cumbersome,

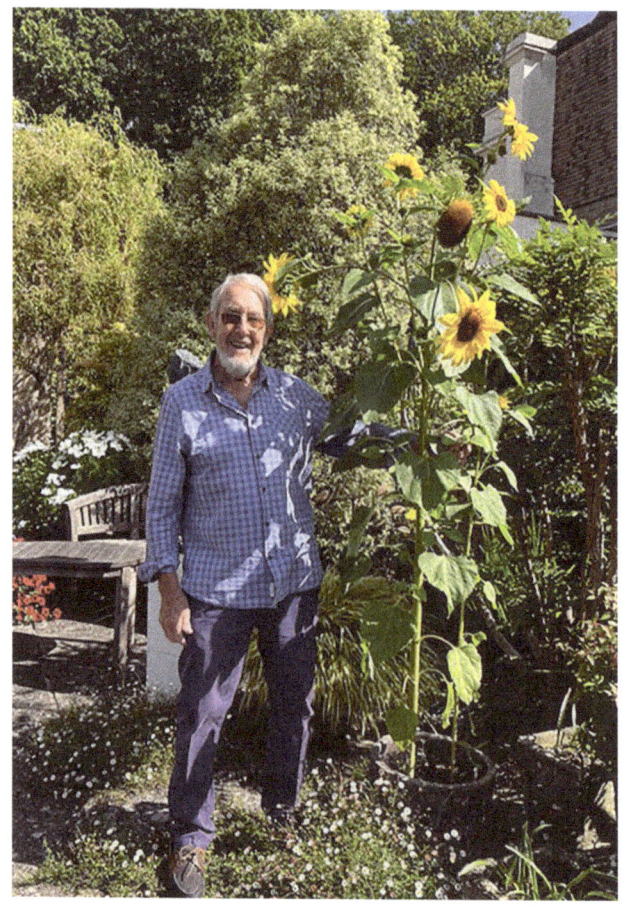

Photo One. LB and sunflowers

oversized, monolithic, unmanageable "super" hospitals to replace our crumbling hospitals[4].

RG's photo of LB with sunflowers to show what she was able to grow from two seeds. These sunflower heads in sunshine are bright and productive – hosting their own local insects and able to receive busy visiting feeders/pollinators, flying and droning between a variety of destinations to promote health and wellbeing! An optimistic and practical demonstration of collaboration and networking of a dispersed service. If you don't believe LB, refer to Vincent Van Gogh – but we all know what happened to him!

---

[4] LB's "cry of the week": a new large hospital has recently opened in the midlands – after "more than a *decade* of collaboration". Started well before Covid came to call this 11-storey facility spans 84,000m^2. It has 700 beds – half are in single rooms. It has 13 operating theatres. Its key architectural intervention is a five-storey internal "winter garden" and has an impressive "accessible roof terrace to promote patient mobility and wellbeing ... offering outdoor spaces for relaxation and reflection", *Architecture Today* newsletter, October 2024. LB, while wishing well to all those that sail in this large new NHS hospital, wonders about the architectural interventions and the patients who may want to get out of this place after day surgery or the shortest possible admission as an inpatient. A quick exit might be a better bet for them to again enjoy being at home and to make use of local community facilities for their wellbeing – perhaps even assisting them with getting back to school, work or retirement in the right frame of mind.

Chapter 1

Dear Mungo and 10,000m² v 90,000m² hospitals

Dear Mungo shone a light from the other side of the planet in August 2024. Mungo is one of the all-time best architects with a keen interest in the design of hospitals. Recently, he has been advising the health service somewhere in Australia about designing a mega "super" hospital of 90,000m² (which is really massive). Why was Mungo doing this, at what cost, who told him to do so and do they really have a clue about the consequences of building such a huge folly?

If anyone can make a mega hospital work, Dear Mungo is the one – but the evidence is stacked against him and he knows it!

Mungo, after dipping into the Dear Susan... sequel, began to wonder about doing a rethink of this current project, but where to start? To begin with, he took great pleasure in assembling, on a large tabletop, a to-scale model of LB's proposed blueprint – a 10,000m² smaller hospital using Lego blocks. He then set this beside a Lego model of his 90,000m² mega hospital. Mungo clearly needed to get his head around why his brief was requiring so much accommodation and such a large pile of Lego!

DEAR MUNGO AND 10,000M² V 90,000M² HOSPITALS

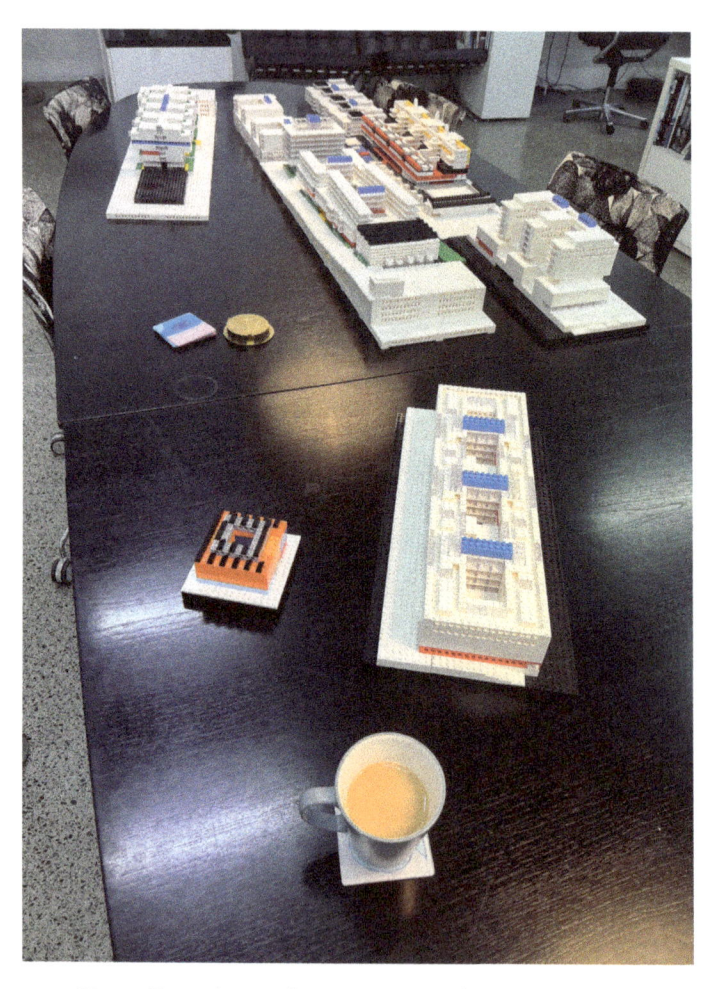

Photo Two shows these two Lego hospital models side by side – one small hospital and one large mega hospital, plus a mug of coffee getting cold. Who in their right mind would think these were interchangeable alternatives? No one, but please read on.

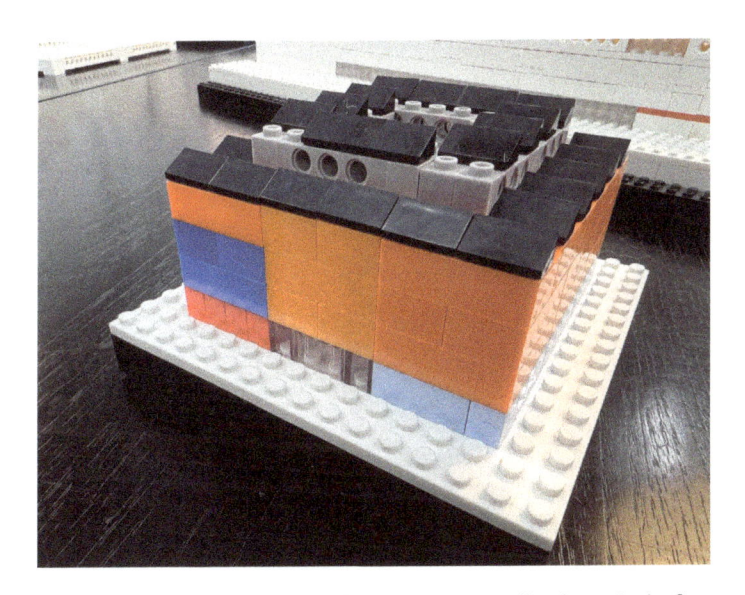

Photo Three shows the four-storey smaller hospital of under 10,000m² including its roofscape. This, to LB, is beginning to look like an efficient, self-sufficient, ready-to-take-on-anything, state-of-the-art tug/hospital of the future – with all guns blazing! Maybe this, because of its implied built-in options/choices, could conceivably become a prototype generic smaller hospital solution for all eventualities – see Chapter 2.

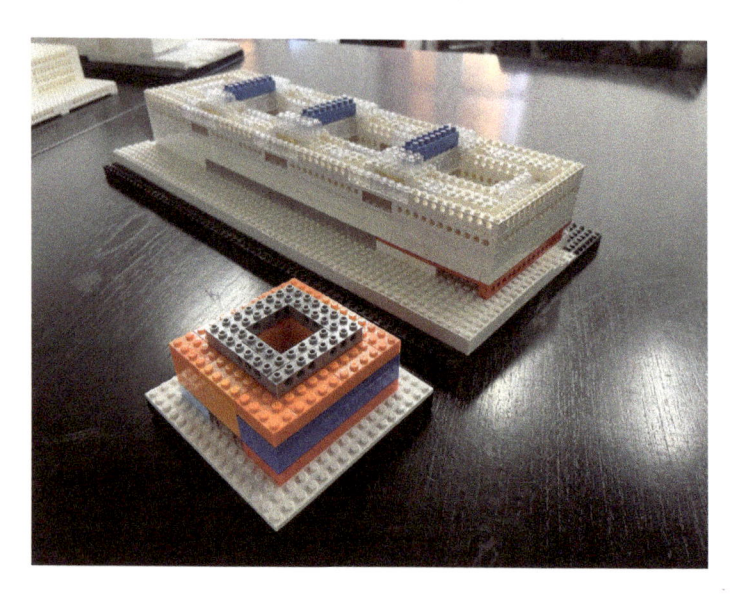

Photo Four shows this "state-of-the-art tug/hospital of the future" looking as if it is coming alongside to assist a potentially obsolete, becalmed, but out of control, 90,000m² mega hospital (in this case a brand new one!). It might be fair to say that a very massive mega hospital might be the ultimate solution for somewhere in Australia with space to build real highways and a population with the energy to travel vast distances for a cure – but a 90,000m² hospital is a massive undertaking if you have got it wrong, cobber!

In the UK, a few new very large hospital developments, planned before Covid, will be completed/funded (hopefully not too many!) to satisfy the political climate. The NHS more likely will be encouraged to try to "transform" parts of those failing large hospitals that need most urgent attention – even when they are beyond being transformable. All large hospitals, whether they are new or transformed, could most certainly do with a "state-of-the-art tug/hospital" to come alongside to save the day.

If those planners somewhere in Australia thought to ask LB (and of course they never would!) what he thought of their plans to centralise all hospital services on one site – a "super" mega state hospital where all state highways lead to hospitalisation – he would have suggested that they should not put all their eggs in one basket case as it would be crazy.

LB would argue, with more than a little supporting evidence, that five or six smaller hospitals of 10,000m² and an allocation of 50,000m²–60,000m² would be sufficient for most services on one site. In limiting the size of this central hospital, demand would soon indicate whether another four or three smaller hospitals of 10,000m² should be provided quickly on the same site as a second stage to meet the anticipated need of 90,000m². If it turned out to be undersized, LB's preference would be to locate the other 30,000–40,000m² off site in a number/variety of locations to better serve local communities.

However, LB would prefer even greater dispersal. Imagine, instead of a soon-to-be-obsolete 90,000m² "super" mega state hospital taking years to plan and construct, a totally dispersed service of six to nine 10,000m² generic smaller hospitals serviced by specialist teams of flying doctors. These teams might arrive as required by air transport or, if need be, patients might be lifted by air ambulance to be flown to where the specialist teams are assembled at any of these smaller hospitals. Networked supplies delivered by drones or fast road transport between each smaller hospital could be coordinated from a central hub arranging for everything from theatre lists to outpatient appointments.

Alternatively, if there really has to be a large hospital to centralise services (the case for which is beyond LB's belief) why not a proposal like the group of smaller hospitals shown in **PLAN X** in the appendix? This shows how five smaller hospitals, designated for different services/users, might fit together on a single site – a worst-case scenario for a single site. It is difficult to imagine this single site with an additional four smaller hospitals in a second stage development alongside a first stage of five smaller hospitals (totalling 90,000m^2).

Ideally, smaller hospitals should be part of a dispersed service using a number of sites. They should be designed to be autonomous and to stand alone wherever/however they are sited – grouped together or sited independently from each other.

The above is about concepts, not details – details are easy!

In order to assist readers of this Dear Susan… paperback (and as discussed in more detail in the first and second versions) smaller hospitals should be:

- Able to be built quickly
- Built and equipped to stand alone, located where they are needed

- Uncomplicated, understandable and flexible
- Therapeutic to inspire confidence
- No larger than 10,000m²
- No higher than four stories high for patient accommodation
- Should have standardised/interchangeable suites, for example theatre suite, X-ray suite, out-patients suite, etc.
- Have less than 100 bedrooms for an inpatient hospital provided with mostly single and some double bedrooms, all with ensuites, except in ITU.
- More like an hotel than a hospital
- Not able to be extended
- Replaced when they become obsolete and as soon as someone thinks about extending them badly
- Accessible by air and road
- Accessible by rail and good public transport or be just around the corner
- Able to provide free and accessible parking – scaled down to suit a productive smaller hospital with high turnover and short-stay events

What the brief for a 90,000m² hospital might ask for is anyone's guess, especially after Covid, and given the size of the waiting list, the state of the crumbling NHS estate, the location of existing hospitals and the bad health of the nation's infrastructure.

Chapter 2
Trauma and Elective Care Centres

Plans are included in this chapter to showcase how new adaptable smaller hospitals might be provided quickly to replace our crumbling failing hospitals. It is thought that smaller hospitals based on these plans might lift morale, renew confidence, and house and promote better services throughout the NHS. The primary aim should be to demonstrate that the NHS will require less beds, not more, by improving performances using the right kind of facilities.

PLAN 7 in the *Dear Susan…* sequel illustrated in small-scale detail the difference between centres for trauma and elective care specialties using a range of options/suites. Trauma was allocated 64 bedrooms and two double operating theatre suites. Whereby, elective care has no bedrooms but two double operating suites and recovery lounges. Both of these centres were shown to be under 10,000m² on four floors.

The following pages in this chapter use enlargements of **PLAN 7** to illustrate how floor plans differ for trauma and elective care centres by setting them side by side and how these can be arranged within the same four-storey building envelope/container.

TRAUMA AND ELECTIVE CARE CENTRES

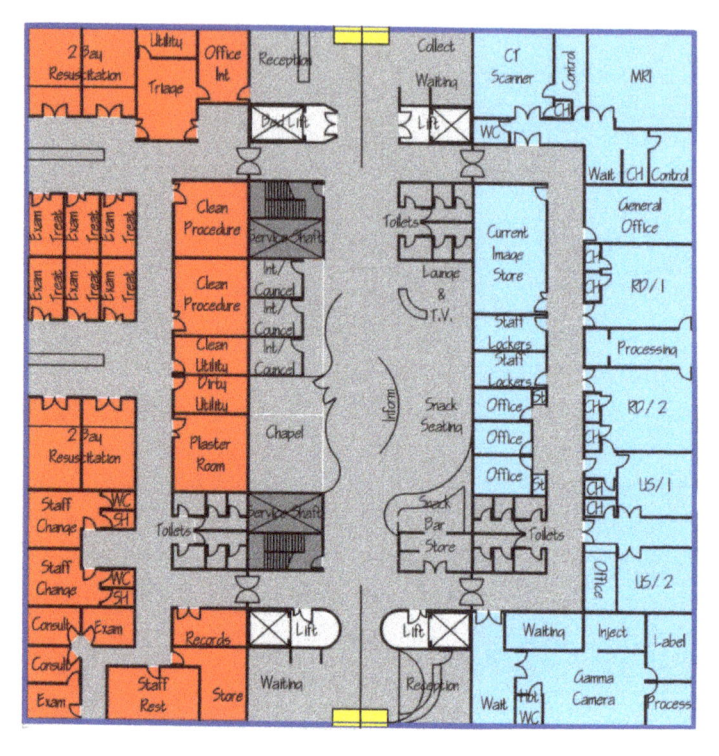

TRAUMA – A/1 (2,250m²)

Main Entrance concourse, major accident suite, X- ray suite with CT and MRI

PLAN A/1 showing a trauma centre – level 0, ground floor

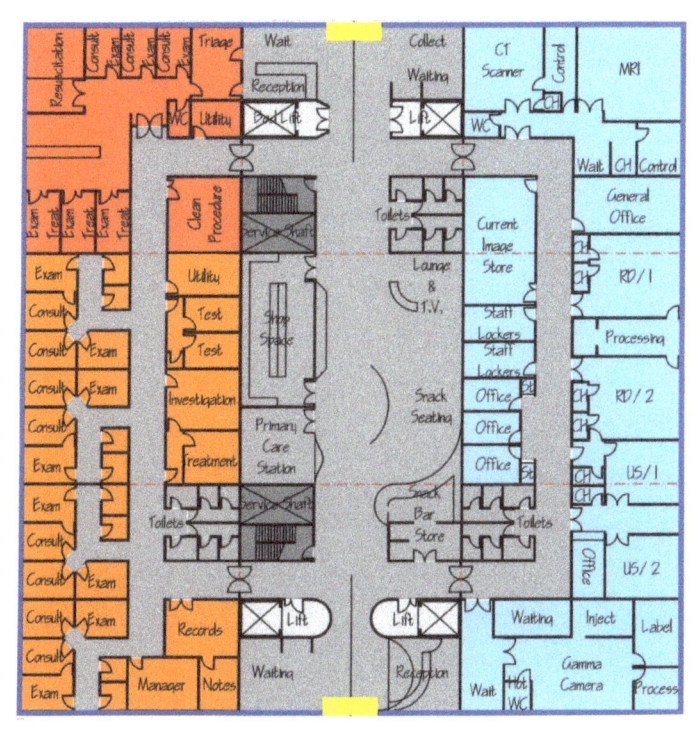

DEAR SUSAN…'LORD D….' & THE GOING DOWN OF THE SUN…

ELECTIVE – B/1 (2,250m²)

Main Entrance concourse, minor accident clinic suite, X-ray suite with CT and MRI, and outpatient suite

PLAN B/1 showing an Elective Care Centre – level 0, ground floor

TRAUMA AND ELECTIVE CARE CENTRES

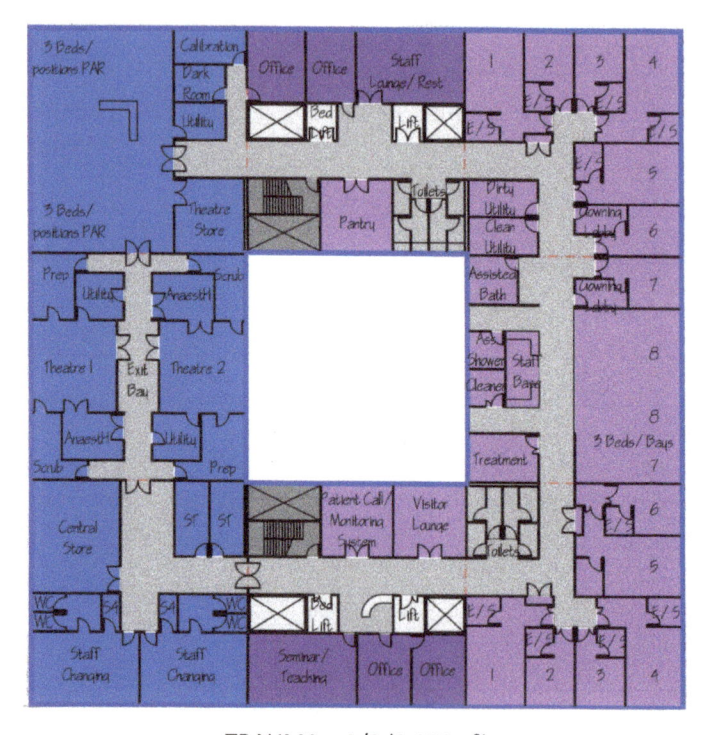

TRAUMA – A/2 (2,000m²)

An operating theatre suite, with two theatres plus PAR and a 16-bed sub-nursing suite
(including a three-bed ITU and a patient monitoring room)
PLAN A/2 showing a trauma centre – level 1, first floor

DEAR SUSAN…'LORD D….' & THE GOING DOWN OF THE SUN…

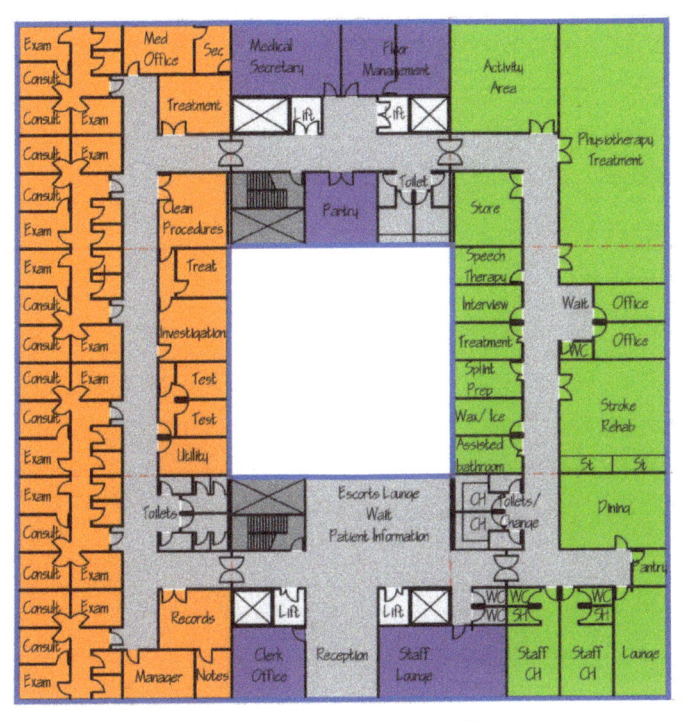

ELECTIVE – B/2 (2,000m²)

Outpatient suite including a mix of consulting, examination and treatment rooms and a rehabilitation suite

PLAN B/2 showing an elective care centre – level 1, first floor

TRAUMA AND ELECTIVE CARE CENTRES

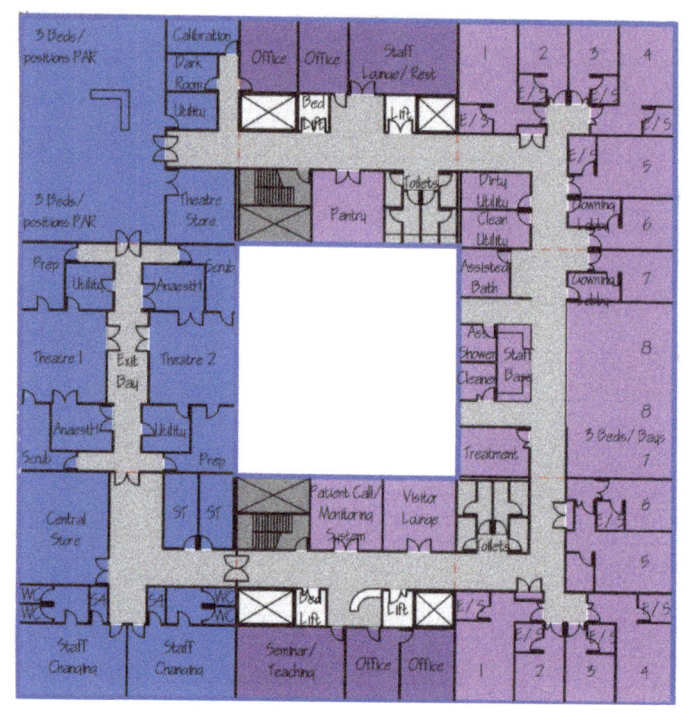

TRAUMA – A/3 (2,000m²)

An operating theatre suite, with two theatres plus PAR and
a 16-bed sub-nursing suite
(including a three-bed ITU and a patient monitoring room)
PLAN A/3 showing a trauma centre – level 2, second floor

DEAR SUSAN…'LORD D….' & THE GOING DOWN OF THE SUN…

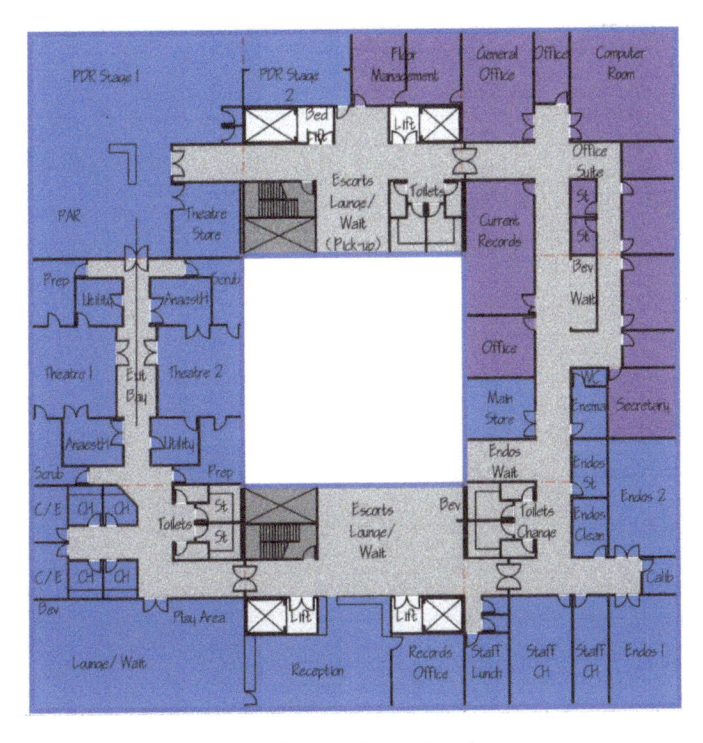

ELECTIVE – B/3 (2,000m²)

Day surgery suite with two operating theatres plus PAR lounges, endoscopy suite and nursing administration suite – note, separate "in and out" routes

PLAN B/3 showing an elective care centre – level 2, second floor

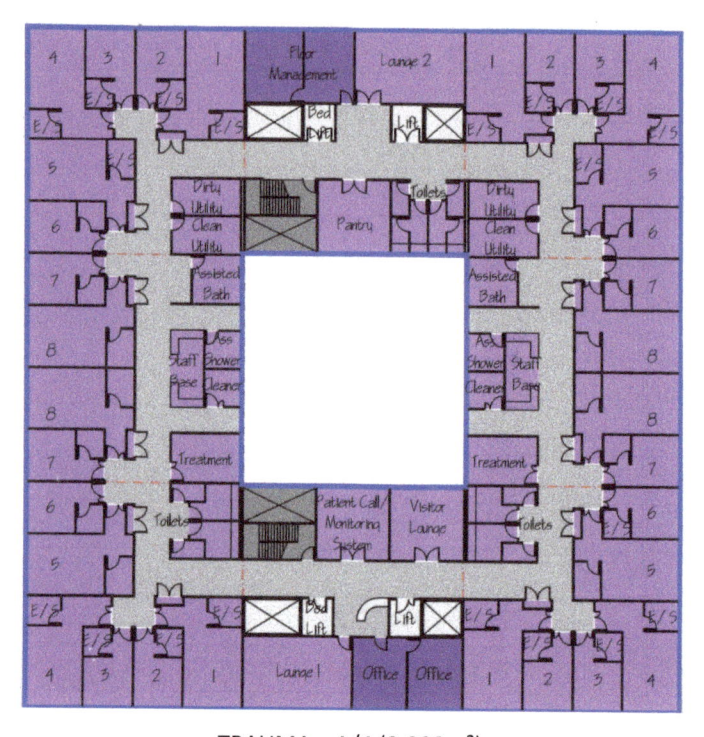

TRAUMA AND ELECTIVE CARE CENTRES

TRAUMA – A/4 (2,000m²)

32 single room ward nursing section in two 16-bed room sub-nursing suites able to be managed as 4 x 8 bed room clusters.

PLAN A/4 showing a trauma centre – level 3, third floor

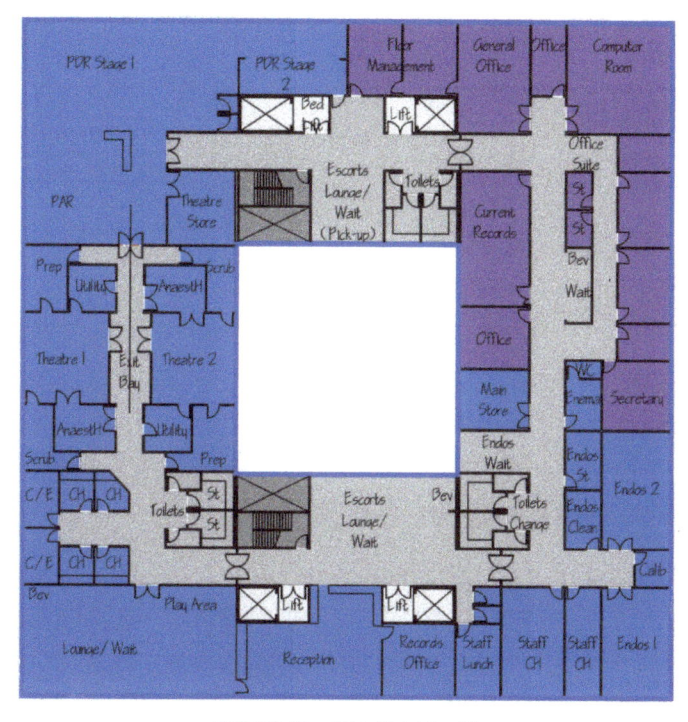

DEAR SUSAN...'LORD D....' & THE GOING DOWN OF THE SUN...

ELECTIVE – B/4 (2,000m²)

Day surgery suite with two operating theatres plus PAR lounges, endoscopy suite and nursing administration suite – note, separate "in and out" routes

PLAN B/4 showing an elective care centre – level 3, third floor.

TRAUMA AND ELECTIVE CARE CENTRES

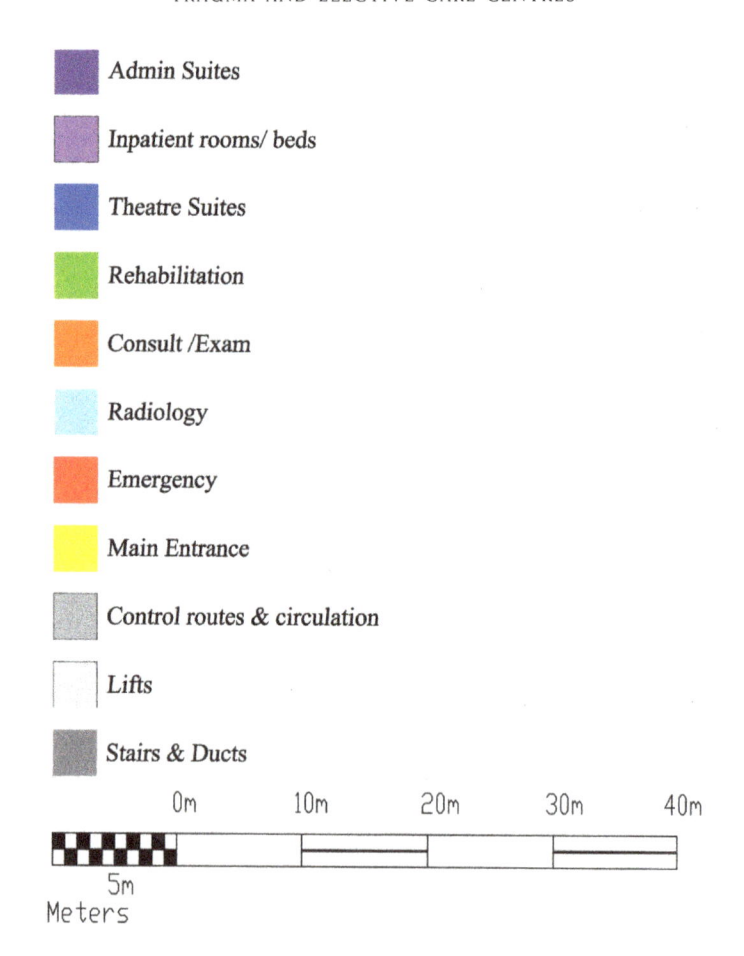

- ■ Admin Suites
- ■ Inpatient rooms/ beds
- ■ Theatre Suites
- ■ Rehabilitation
- ■ Consult /Exam
- ■ Radiology
- ■ Emergency
- ■ Main Entrance
- ■ Control routes & circulation
- □ Lifts
- ■ Stairs & Ducts

0m   10m   20m   30m   40m

5m
Meters

Colour key and scale for Plans in Chapter 2

These are included for readers who might find these useful for getting to understand the coloured plans in this chapter in more detail.

Readers of the first *Dear Susan...* paperback were not able to look at architectural plans illustrating smaller hospitals. This was because LB had found over many years that people best placed to change policy and implement new strategies for the NHS tended to turn a blind eye at the sight of a plan or drawing. This was no matter how diagrammatic or coloured up a presentation or how enthusiastic the presenter. It is therefore hardly surprising that the NHS is struggling with a crumbling estate. With this in mind, here are a few more "words" to supplement the above plans if they are too difficult to understand.

In choosing to construct smaller hospitals, these must not only be small but must also be affordable, secure, uncomplicated, understandable, flexibly and intensively used and changeable without needing structural refits that might mean closing the hospital. They should also be inspiring, and because of all these qualities, healing.

A trauma centre would be "open all hours" and be planned as shown above with suites for emergency admissions/triage, scanners/X-rays, two-times-two operating theatre suites (with PAR) and inpatient bedrooms. It should be self-sufficient and able to stand alone. It is shown to have a total of 64 bedrooms, in two wards of 32 single and double bedrooms. These are shown to divide into 16-bedroom sub-nursing suites dividable into eight-bed room clusters for treating trauma and the long road to recovery.

These eight-bedroom clusters might be allocated for high and medium dependency or women only, men only, children, older people, specialist treatment groups or allocated randomly.

Trauma centres might be located where they are needed – not necessarily on an existing hospital site – if possible along and around motorways and connected by air ambulance and fast road ambulance services.

The elective care centre, being a day surgery facility, would be open from 7am 'til midnight. It would be planned and equipped with suites for reception, consultation/treatment, scanners/X-ray, two-times-two operating theatre suites, recovery lounges and a rehabilitation suite. Inpatient accommodation will not be provided. These centres would be totally self-sufficient for day surgery procedures.

Elective care centres could be located alongside trauma centres or be sited to be more accessible for local communities, if necessary on an existing hospital site but self-contained.

The Grid Plan below shows that circulation is via a racetrack return corridor from lift to lift and stair to stair. Please note the "drop-off" and "pick-up" points. It is intended that from receptions on the ground floor – level 0, patients will be directed from the public areas in the main entrance concourse to the appropriate suite and the nearest lift to patient facilities on the upper floors. Lifts would be monitored on all levels. Patient flows are straightforward throughout each suite. The comfort, privacy, and security of people using these smaller hospitals would be safeguarded as they move up through each level from the public spaces on the ground floor, level 0 to the treatment and therapy spaces at intermediate levels and finally, in the case of an inpatient centre, up through to the private hotel standard single

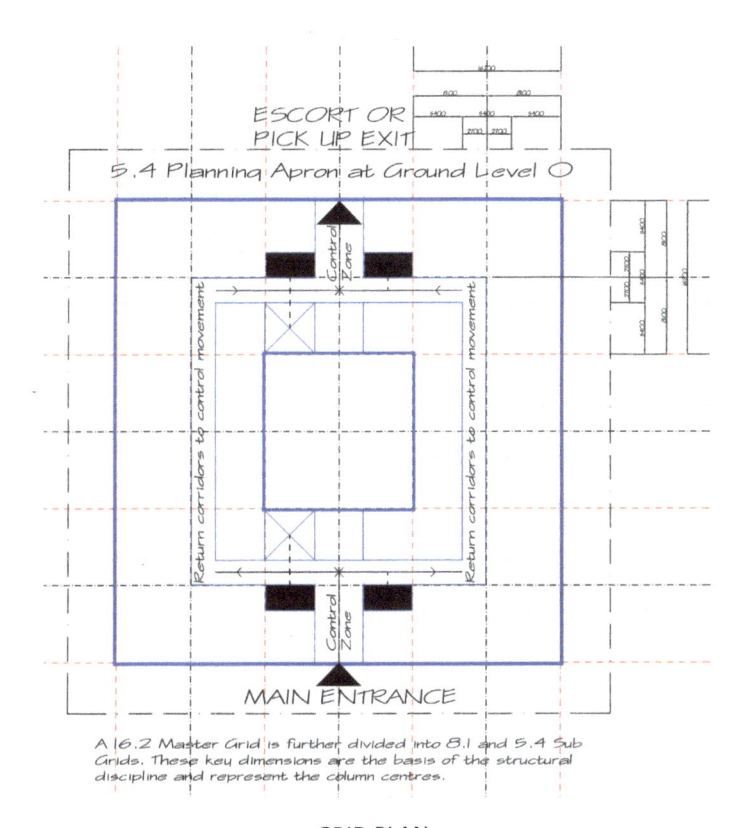

[Figure: Grid Plan diagram showing Main Entrance, Escort or Pick Up Exit, Control Zones, Return corridors to control movement, and annotation "5.4 Planning Apron at Ground Level O". Caption below: "A 16.2 Master Grid is further divided into 8.1 and 5.4 Sub Grids. These key dimensions are the basis of the structural discipline and represent the column centres."]

GRID PLAN

and double bedrooms on the upper levels. More detail is shown in **Plans A/1 – A/4** and **B/1 – B/4**.

LB would hope that these trauma and elective care centres would be bright, shiny, optimistic, and therapeutic machines for healing – full of hope and promise. Less staff would be doing much more to mend/cure any condition/symptom and reduce the need for lengthy hospital admissions. A quick turnround of patients and a community support network with direct communications to these smaller hospitals would put right without fuss any mishap on a journey to a full recovery.

It is difficult to leave this chapter without further "words" to describe TRAUMA – **PLANS A/2, A/3** and **A/4** and without drawing the reader's attention to the ward layouts illustrated. These layouts show how the NHS might take "a leap in the dark" to make smaller hospitals work for patients.

A 32-bedroom ward and a 16-bedroom sub-nursing suite

A 32-bedroom ward suite is divided into two 16-bedroom sub-nursing suites and further divided to provide four eight-bedroom clusters. These eight-bedroom clusters might be allocated for specialist treatment groups, high dependency patients, medium dependency step-down, women only, men only, children, older people or allocated randomly.

There is a mix of single and double-size bedrooms each with an ensuite. The double- size bedrooms are to allow a spouse/partner/carer to stay with an adult patient needing assistance or a parent to stay with an unwell child or to allow a patient requiring a longer length of stay to have a comfortable "place like home"

Each 16-bedroom sub-nursing suite has a patient lounge, a nursing station, an assisted bathroom and shower and treatment/utility rooms. Partitioning to form the three bedrooms opposite the nursing station can be dismantled to form a three-bed ITU when combined with an operating suite as a step-down from PAR – see **PLAN A/2, A/3** and **A/4**.

The 32-bedroom ward has a patient monitoring room, a visitors lounge and pantry to distribute an appetising choice of meals – see **PLAN A/4**.

Chapter 3
So, what about other specialties?

Chapter 2 sets out the difference between a trauma centre and an elective care centre. These two specialties were chosen to show how smaller hospitals can be radically different from each other and from old-style district general hospitals. Hopefully these plans might help buck the trend for developing larger, super mega hospitals. Also, more importantly after Covid, smaller hospital like those illustrated are urgently required now to resuscitate the NHS to get it up and running again.

Trauma and elective care centres are shown to be accommodated in the same for-storey envelope/ container or "box" having been allocated different suites to meet different functions. For example, trauma is shown to have 64 bedrooms and elective care no inpatient beds at all. So, if need be, the same four-storey envelope/container of 8,250m² (less than the maximum of 10,000m²), allowing for choices/selections/options, might be used to provide smaller hospitals for a wide range of specialties like emergency care, cancer care, chronic care, care of older people if there is a gap in these services and are seen to be a priority.

SO, WHAT ABOUT OTHER SPECIALTIES?

For example, with reference to the PLANS used in Chapter 2, the following specialties might stack up as follows:

Level	*Women and Children*	*Community Care*	*Renal Care*
Level 3	PLAN A/4	PLAN A/4	PLAN A/4
Level 2	PLAN A/3	PLAN B/3	PLAN A/2
Level 1	PLAN B/2	PLAN B/2	PLAN B/2[5]
Level 0	PLAN B/1	PLAN B/1	PLAN B/1

Colours are used on the plans in Chapter 2 to show how mix-and-match suites are arranged for the two illustrated specialties of trauma and elective care. These mix-and-match suites range from 250m² for a minor injury clinic up to 2,000m² for a 32-bedroom ward – these suites are illustrated in PLAN C:

---

[5] An outpatient suite would be exchanged for a renal dialysis suite on level 1.

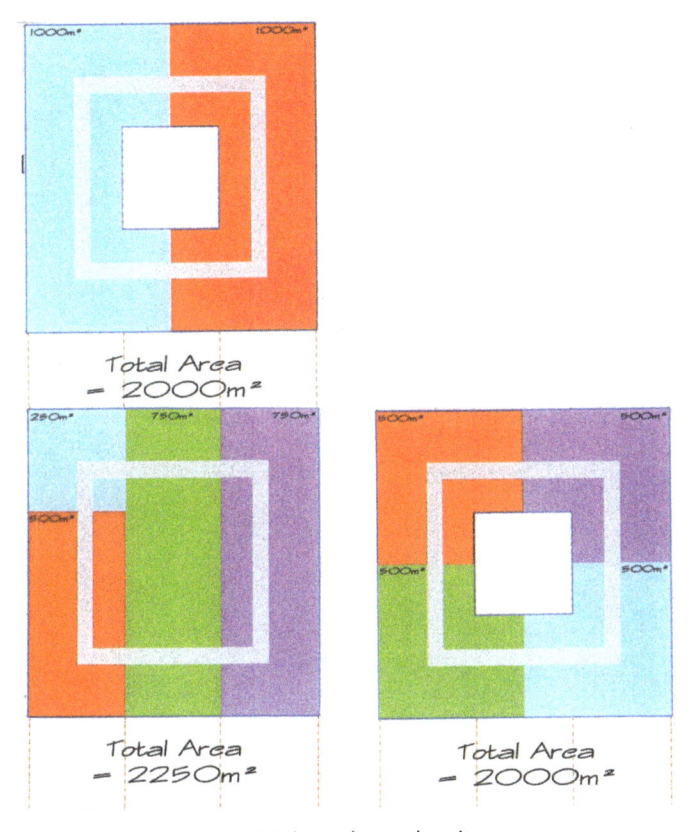

PLAN C Mix-and-match suites

These suites are interchangeable in relation to the specialties selected for a smaller hospital. Suites have already been selected/allocated for the trauma care and elective care centres illustrated in Chapter 2. However, a local NHS might prefer a different selection as show in **PLAN D** below. This cut and paste plan shows how a local preference to have all four operating theatres at the same level might be arranged.

SO, WHAT ABOUT OTHER SPECIALTIES?

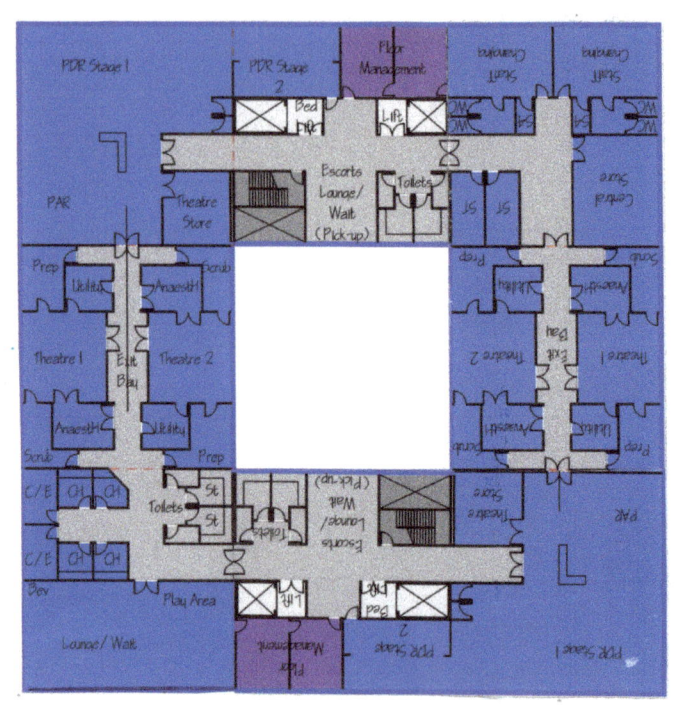

PLAN D (2,000m²), a mix-and-match variation

Two 1,000m² operating theatre suites, each with two (a pair) theatres plus PAR side-by-side on the same level/floor

Chapter 4
May the four-storey limit be exceeded?

Yes, in cities and towns it might have to be exceeded but LB hopes that the criteria set out in Chapter 1 for a smaller hospital can still be met. Plans used in Chapter 2 have been tinkered with to illustrate how two four-storey smaller hospitals might be stacked, one on top of the other, and be managed separately.

PLANS E and **F** below show that by inserting an additional 5.4 metre slice of extra accommodation on both sides of the square plan it would be possible to increase/stretch the size of the square light well to form a rectangle. This extra space might be used to introduce two more banks of non-stop lifts travelling from levels/floors 0-4 and from there serving each level/floor from 4-7 and the roof space.

This tinkering shows that a local NHS, if able to make a case for providing a trauma and elective care combination to replace part of a failing hospital on a small urban site, might consider such a proposal.

What is important here is that when stacked the two centres should be managed separately as self-sufficient

MAY THE FOUR-STOREY LIMIT BE EXCEEDED?

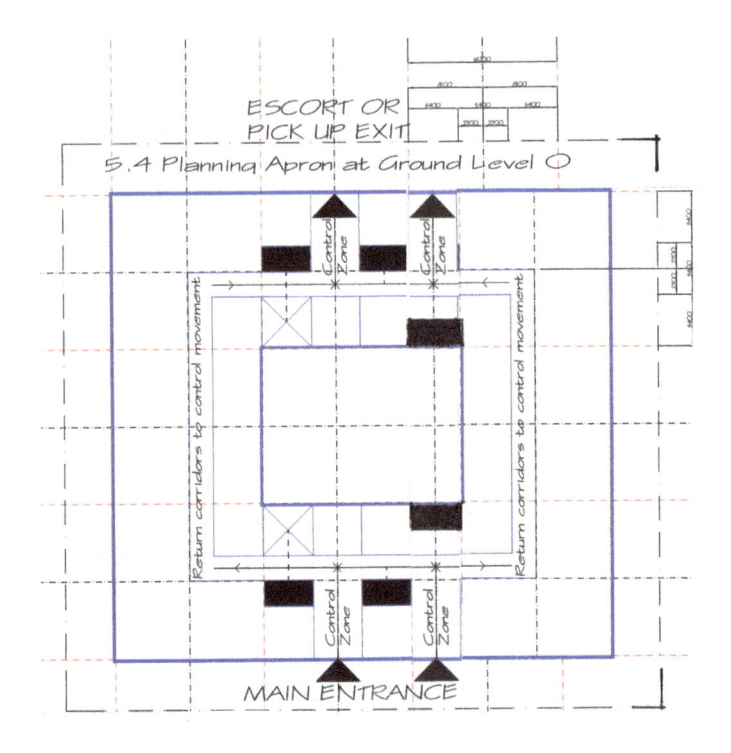

PLAN E

Showing the planning grid extended by inserting an additional 5.4 metre slice on both sides of the square – if two four-storey smaller hospitals are stacked.

trauma and elective care centres. However, there is no reason why both centres cannot share the extended level 0/ground floor main entrance concourse when all patients, their visitors, and staff from both centres want a snack or have a need to pray – see **PLAN F**.

The choice is yours to decide which centre is stacked on top of the other, but LB thinks trauma should take the lower four storeys as it will be "open all hours" to take

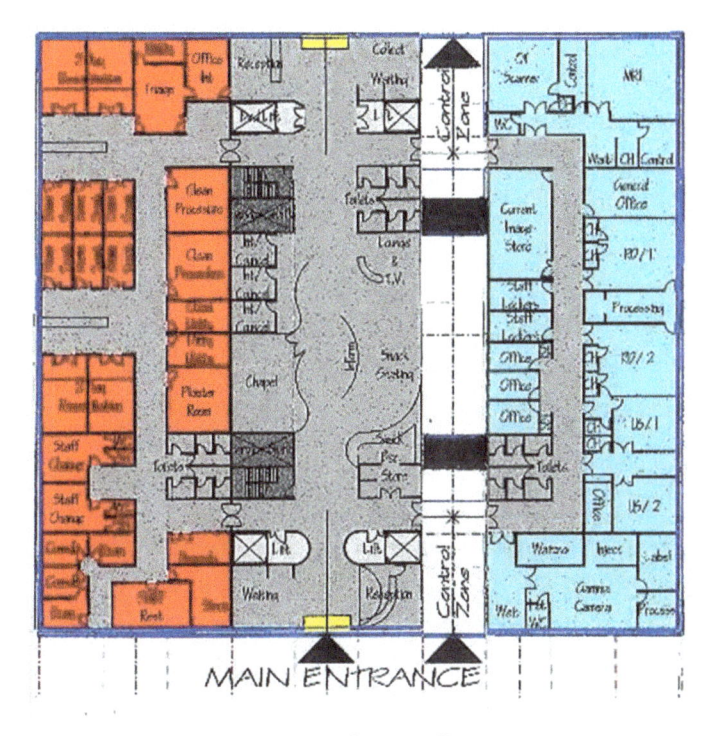

PLAN F (2,500m²)

Showing an extended ground floor for a stacked trauma centre/ elective care centre – at level 0 – for comparison also see PLAN A/1 in Chapter 2

emergencies. The four-storey elective care centre on top will open 7am 'til midnight and close during the early hours.

LB has found, during his struggles to describe smaller hospitals for his lay target audience via an easy read paperback, that something can turn up to spark off a sentence or two or more! His fall from grace requiring emergency hospital services during the first year of Covid in November 2020 sparked off the first 'Dear Susan...'

paperback published in July 2023. The lack of responses from his target audience to this first Dear Susan... led to its sequel published in May 2024 and then 'Lord D....' came to call in November 2024 to steer this third paperback.

An article in the RIBA Journal of January 2025 has usefully helped LB to slightly extend this chapter. This article 'Box Clever' describes the design of a speculative office block in Paddington designed by Renzo Piano the architect for the Shard.

If you need a 'real model' to understand how a smaller hospital 'stacked' to combine Trauma and Elective Care Centres might fit onto a site in a congested part of London, you might hot foot it to Paddington Square off Praed Street. This 18-storey square box office block sits on a site vacated by the Royal Mail, whose sorting office was demolished to make way. It is set between "Brunel's Paddington Station and the rambling St. Mary's Hospital complex. The 55 metres by 55 metres box (footprint) is set high with two levels of retail and a London Underground Station beneath". It has the same footprint as the 'GRID PLAN' included in Chapter 2.

Had the developer knocked on St. Mary's door to propose building a machine for healing the NHS instead of an office block leased to an investment fund manager, St. Mary's might have been in a position to face an optimistic future. With its own underground station beneath and a helicopter pad at roof level, this might have been a perfect fit to provide improved health care services to the local community and beyond.

For the curious, had this knock on the door happened, the Trauma Centre might reasonably have been stacked on top of the Elective Care Centre. This would allow easy access for patients arriving at roof top level by air ambulance. Rapid rise lifts external to the building would bring emergency patients arriving by road ambulance directly to the major accident suite triage. Elective day patients could walk to Paddington Square or arrive at the entrance to the lower Elective Care Centre using the underground beneath, train, bus, taxi or bicycle – with little or no need for car parking.

Perhaps in time, as the need for office space continues to diminish, this clever box might become vacant to be refitted by Renzo Piano with the help of Dear Mungo for a forward-thinking NHS, having swapped redundant parts of the rambling St. Mary's Hospital complex with the same developer – pigs might fly!

Chapter 5

Reasons offered up for doing nothing!

The most worrying aspect of LB's message proposing that the NHS might be provided with new smaller hospitals quickly, is that the target audience listed in this Dear Susan... paperback's introduction has little or no view in support of this blueprint.

An obvious reason for doing little or nothing after Covid is that there is no money available given the state of the public finances. Not even the money previously promised during the Covid pandemic to "build 40 new hospitals".

Or, "larger hospitals have better outcomes" – which is difficult to get your head around when the waiting list for surgical or medical procedures tops seven million unwell people!

Or, "he is devoting more time to foreign affairs" – which admittedly is a fair point when the many conflicts across the world must be a worthy priority.

Or, settling the pay of junior doctors – clearly one of life's imponderables settled for now by a 22.3% pay rise.

REASONS OFFERED UP FOR DOING NOTHING!

Or, a priority being given to recruitment and training – another one of life's imponderables especially hand-in-hand with a built-in brain drain for working abroad when fully trained because of the awful working conditions over here.

Or, a total denial about the state of the NHS infrastructure and how this is a straight-jacket for the continuing development of the NHS – that is until Lord Darzi identified "crumbling buildings" as an obstruction to change. Also, coming to terms with the colossal backlog maintenance costs, which if ever funded is always likely to be money badly spent.

Or, a hope that private health care (which is always provided in hospitals smaller than those provided for the NHS and often in buildings looking and feeling more like hotels with capacity to see more NHS patients than it currently does) might in our lifetime take over responsibility for the health of the nation – at least for those in a position to pay for health care in a two- tier service.

Or, that people are opposed in principle to "standard" solutions for a uniform and fair NHS.

Or, sadly that the architectural profession is hell-bent on making sure that each new project is an original design concept – which is fine if seeking the truth is really more important than reducing the waiting list and dealing with the health and well-being of the population.

Or, worst of all, apathy or buck-passing! "I would suggest that you raise this issue directly with your own MP as it is a local issue"

And so on! including the non- building initiatives being implemented currently like NHS diagnostic centres, virtual wards and surgical hubs. These have a greater emphasis on care in the community using existing facilities along with "social prescribing" initiatives.

Given that there seems to be plenty of reasons offered up for doing nothing and not delivering smaller hospitals quickly, are there any reasons for doing so?

'Lord D....' (flagged-up on this *Dear Susan...* front cover) is of course Lord Darzi. His rapid investigation of the state of the NHS had much to say, but not a lot about the kind of hospitals needed to change the state of the NHS estate. Clearly, Lord Darzi has many other causes for concern, having reported that the NHS is in serious trouble. Even he admits that "the sheer scope of issues facing the health service, however, has been hard to quantify and articulate." Even with his cast of hundreds (maybe thousands), Lord Darzi is suggesting that improving the NHS will take time. "It has taken more than a decade for the NHS to fall into disrepair ... But it will take years rather than months to get the health service back to peak performance ... it is unlikely that waiting lists can be cleared and other performance standards restored in one parliamentary term"

Whilst LB appreciates Lord Darzi's point that it has taken more than a decade for the NHS to fall into disrepair, does it really have to take another 10 years to put it right?

Lord Darzi's review is available for all to read including his major themes for the forth coming ten-year health plan. Key pointers for LB's message are:

- The NHS Has been starved of capital – it has "crumbling" buildings.
- There is a shortfall of £37 billion of capital investment.
- The NHS budget is not being spent where it should be – too greater a share is being spent on hospitals.
- The NHS is in a critical condition but its vital signs are strong.
- Too many staff are disengaged.
- A&E is in an awful state.
- Waiting times have ballooned.
- The picture on quality of care is mixed.
- And last but not least – the patients' voice is not loud enough.

Might not new smaller hospitals be part of the answer? The aim should be to reduce admissions to as short a period as possible. Better hospitals with the latest no-expense-spared equipment could help increase the turnover of patients using staff already in the NHS to improve outcomes. *New smaller hospitals should be built to help save lives.*

Everything about the NHS is too big to handle. It is time to downsize so all users can feel part of something tangible, which might help to restore confidence in the NHS.

A reason for doing something?

After the very worst of Covid, the NHS must now deal with a constant flow of emergencies and a massive backlog of less urgent but significant injuries and illnesses that are crippling the population. A different strategy should be tried. This could provide a rapidly built new generation of trauma and elective care centres. Also, it could eventually provide a range of rapidly built centres like those for accident/emergency, women and children, cancer care, renal care, chronic care, care of older people and rehabilitation and so on in new, fast, easy, smart, smaller hospitals. However, the immediate need is for trauma and elective care surgical centres. These can be built to sidestep what went before and what is going on now to inappropriately transform larger failing older hospitals, many of which are of the wrong time and are now in the wrong place. All specialities other than trauma and elective care could continue to use suitable and better maintained existing hospitals like the last generation of nucleus hospitals until they also need replacing with new smaller hospitals

In a nutshell, NHS staff have the skills needed and there are probably enough of them trained up and ready to start all over again even though many feel that they have had enough. However, most of the time they have the wrong vehicle to change speed, break new ground and to help drive forward a new strategy.

Chapter 6
Smaller Hospitals should be...?

After Covid, surely we have gone beyond the days of long-term planning cycles and drawn-out public consultations leading only to gradual and begrudging ways to improve redundant hospitals. Or worse, to the provision of monolithic, inflexible new super mega hospitals that are guaranteed to become a burden for decades. We must urgently change this mindset.

It is hoped that readers are able to absorb the essential details on the coloured plans used in Chapter 2. From these it should be possible to understand the proposed content on each level/floor of two four-story smaller hospitals, specialising in trauma and elective care. These plans use a total of 8,250m² from an allocation/limit of 10,000m². Subject to location, it is assumed that a contingency allocation of 1,750m² might be used for local add-ons if needed, like pathology, pharmacy or any other service not readily available nearby. This contingency is more likely to be taken up by a trauma care centre because ideally it is likely to stand alone in its own war zone and a much wider catchment area taking in a number of counties. It is because of its specialisation it might be located near motorways, and airports on the edge of or apart from the number of built-up areas it is serving. An elective care centre should ideally be sited within its community and consideration might be given to "sharing" local enterprises and resources.

Local services that might be available nearby for a smaller hospital to tap into might include chemist shops, supermarkets, nurseries, well-being clinics offering yoga therapy, acupuncture, reflexology, massage, etc, keep-fit centres to aid rehabilitation and fitness, as has always been done for chiropody, primary care and funeral services. This could allow smaller NHS hospitals to be "stripped down" to focus on its business of healing with well-being and continuing support handed to but co-ordinated with nearby community services.

Likewise, perhaps it is now time to offload carparking responsibilities to local authorities or private providers especially in built up areas. **PLAN X** in the Appendix shows five smaller hospitals grouped on a single site. It also shows how much space is often taken up for parking when provided by the NHS for patients, visitors and staff on the site of a larger hospital of over 200 beds. It is time that the NHS stopped having a need to buy up land for carparking for larger hospitals. This might be helped by building smaller hospitals that are more part of the community fabric with speedy boarding and a rapid through-put leading to a radically different demand for carparking – this surely must make sense?

LB's attempt at a blueprint for the NHS in this third Dear Susan... paperback encourages a move away from larger, super, mega hospitals and to provide smaller hospitals of less than 10,000m². It also shows how these might take up as little as 8,250m² if they could plug in to local services. So, how small are smaller hospitals able to get and are there sites available in the community?

Over the last 20 years robot-assisted surgery has been developing at pace. We are now hearing about robots assisting transplant operations in the United States. Minimally invasive robotic surgery using systems like the Da Vinci Xi are reducing drastically the length of stay in hospitals to days rather than weeks for complex procedures – so why are we maintaining/retaining all these hospital beds of the wrong type?

Interestingly, a walk about our towns might provide part of the answer to these questions given that high streets are emptying and our shopping habits are changing. For example, in Dorking, the largest and most impressive buildings have been left empty after all the high street banks jumped on the band wagon and left town, followed by the Post Office and the Royal Mail. More interestingly, in Guildford, Debenhams and The House of Fraser have also packed their bags and its two shopping malls are looking underused and vulnerable. Would the Centre Court shopping mall in Wimbledon or Bentall/Fenwick's in Kingston move over for the NHS?

For the time being, LB will stick with his definition of smaller hospitals and continue to promote their construction under a new hospital-buildings-led initiative. The conversion of shopping malls may come later. However, if the NHS is able to bring systems like Da Vinci Xi on stream over the next 10 years he would reconsider reducing the number of bedrooms in the trauma care centre illustrated in Chapter 2 by half - omitting the 32-bedroom ward on Level 3!

Chapter 7

Next Steps?

Readers are allowed to skip this chapter or bin this paperback if they already know the answers for sorting out the NHS. Maybe they, whoever they might be, will share their thoughts in the proposed ten-year plan when it is published in the spring of 2025. However, LB, whoever he might be, feels a need to regurgitate parts of the first and second Dear Susan… paperbacks as a means of summarising what the next steps might be, or should be, in order to start to provide smaller hospital quicky.

On 31st October, the government announced its plans for the NHS, including new money amounting to 1.57 billion for new surgical hubs, scanners and radiotherapy machines *"to double the number of diagnostic scanners with AI enabled technology – meaning less staff would be needed to diagnose illnesses"*. The government's overall pledge is to increase the number of NHS appointments and procedures in England by 40,000 per week.

This is looking a bit like "new wine in old bottles". Surely we should be spending some of this allocation on new "bottles" too? Especially where these might alleviate the pain caused by those many crumbling hospitals that nowadays are often in the wrong place[6].

The first and second Dear Susan… paperbacks set out a submission sent by LB and RG to the Health and Social Care Committee dated 3rd September 2021. This included a road map to show how adaptable, new, smaller hospitals could be provided quickly to replace our many failing hospitals. The following paragraphs revisit this submission as time has been lost since the Covid pandemic, in holding a general election and while the new government puts its feet under the table.

Lord Darzi's report has triggered action from the treasury but it is looking like the NHS will have to struggle on until the spring 2025 to understand the extent of the new ten-year plan. However, the recent flurry of activity confirms the government's determination to drastically improve the performance of the NHS and hopefully to try to get to grips with the state of the NHS estate.

With this in mind it might be worth summarising what the previous chapters of this third paperback are suggesting followed by a revised road map for achieving this kind of proposal

New smaller hospitals should be in the right location, probably sited away from, but used in conjunction

---

[6] It seems highly unlikely that those newspeak "turnaround teams" and "top performers" will achieve much in crumbling hospital buildings. Also, putting new AI scanners in old bottles does sound crazy to some of us – especially if it extends the life of the existing crumbling buildings!

with, an existing hospital, be assembled quickly, be affordable within a fixed capital cost, up to 10,000m² in size and have more relevance to the way surgical teams will have to work in the future. They should also be uncomplicated, patient-friendly, therapeutic, flexible, intensively used and be a key part of a community health and wellbeing service – a machine for healing.

Now is the time to showcase how new, adaptable, smaller hospitals can be provided quickly to replace our many crumbling failing hospitals.

If our government is really interested in recognising how much the NHS estate and its existing hospital buildings are straightjacketing innovation and evolving services and a real need to meet current and emerging challenges, here is a tentative road map:

1. Department of Health and Social Care/NHS to appoint a "turnaround" control team to set up parameters (a prototype) for a network of new, smaller hospitals and a "top performer" to project manage a first wave.
2. Invite top performers in local NHS trusts to apply to be selected to build a new, smaller trauma or elective care centre (or another specialist centre if there is a demand and is already under consideration).
3. Set up a selection process focussing on the following: their proposals to deal with the waiting list; thoughts on managing staff cohesion; how they can demonstrate achieving an improved performance from new facilities; their thoughts

on a potential site and the suitability of its location; are they ready and able to move quickly to build and commission a new facility and how they intend to manage vacated premises.
4. When selected each new smaller hospital project should be monitored and evaluated to report on performance and outcomes.

In working towards the production of brand new, smaller hospitals to kick-start a revitalised hospital construction programme, it should be noted that stockpiles of data and guidance exist which could be utilised to inform how new smaller hospitals might be planned, designed and commissioned. Solutions used in this paperback are based on this wealth of information. Furthermore, Architects for Health, a special interest group affiliated to the RIBA, could apply its expertise in sourcing data and overseeing the early development stages of the road map[7]. If they were to join forces with an enthusiastic DHSC/NHS control team, together they could set parameters for a first wave of smaller hospitals. This control team could quickly assess applicants, ratify the planning and design, be involved as necessary with the manufacture/construction process and when operational monitor and compare performance.

---

[7] There are some architectural practices bursting to design a high-tech futures hospital. Some, after leading their field internationally, have never been commissioned to design a relevant, ground-breaking healthcare building for the NHS (like Rogers, Foster, Hadid and Grimshaw). What a difference these and some of the bright, younger practices might make given half a chance to help design a first wave/network of smaller hospitals.

Chapter 8

A machine for healing?

At the Labour Party Conference in September 2024, the Secretary of State for Health and Social Care told delegates:

> "I know the doctor's diagnosis can sometimes be hard to bear. But if you don't have an accurate diagnosis, you won't provide the correct prescription. And when you put protecting the reputation of the NHS above protecting patients, you're not helping the NHS, you're killing it with kindness."
>
> 25th September 2024

This Secretary of State's ten-year plan, expected in the spring of 2025, will indicate whether this is just political mumbo jumbo or a call for action. It will be interesting to know if he and his advisers can get around to doing something for the NHS and its patients and staff by prioritising the construction of a few smaller hospitals quickly. Certainly, change must be forthcoming to get to grips with the healthcare needs of our population.

On the 13th November 2024, Wes Streeting promised a ***"no holds-barred sweeping review"*** of NHS performance in England. Hospitals can be expected to be ranked on indicators such as care delivery and finances, so patients can see whether they are receiving a good service! And *"turnaround teams"* will be sent into struggling trusts, while *"top performers"* will have more freedom over spending.

We are told that top performers will be given more capital and greater control over where to invest it – be that new equipment or technology or modernising their buildings.

It would be wonderful if architects and engineers could be encouraged by these "top performers" to design smaller hospitals that are truly therapeutic, uplifting and informative. These should house a responsive and enthusiastic service for all patients. It should be clear to patients, as soon as they walk in or are carried through its doors that that a quick procedure is available in a caring, comfortable and positive place. A kind of Holy Grail challenge, to provide smaller hospitals quickly which are transparent and as obvious as a car wash which is fully understandable once you have posted your token and shut your window[8]

Imagine, arriving or being delivered to a stand-alone trauma centre, reaching out to put a gold or silver token in a slot as you enter – when treatment is most needed. After walking or being assisted through on a walk-in/travellator scanner for an automatic triage/diagnosis (a better, more sophisticated piece of apparatus than the

---

[8] This analogy was first enjoyed by LB and Archie McNab (his tutor) in the 1970s – it has been a long time coming!

security screening portal and baggage X-ray machine that we now experience at airports when moving through to the departure lounge), your AI-monitored condition alerts the appropriate specialist team so that you can be dealt with urgently and efficiently and be allowed to leave as soon as you get a green light. On leaving, even if this means a short stopover in an upper floor single bedroom or adjacent motel/healthcare hotel, you should be totally cleansed of all blemishes. You will have got the measure of the place, understood the processes, be thankful for the reliability of staff and equipment, feel optimistic, be done and dusted and fit for the long road ahead!

Hey Ho! This may be pure fantasy but the pattern book of plans included in the Dear Susan… sequel and in this third paperback are derivatives of the plans and data illustrated in the many publications describing the nucleus design and briefing system. However, these plans, in showing how to move a step forward towards promoting and illustrating smaller hospitals are a darn sight nearer to showing what a healing machine might look like. More so, than the development of super mega hospitals, with far too many beds, in overblown restrictive institutions which are a move in the wrong direction if we are serious about sorting out the NHS estate and in revitalising its service to all patients.

Rachel Power, the chief executive of the Patients Association was quoted as saying in response to the 13th November 2024 announcements:

"We hope trusts who receive greater funding freedom will use this money wisely – to cut waiting times, make

the waiting experience better for patients and strengthen the ways they work with patients to improve services."

In this third Dear Susan... paperback, nucleus hospitals data has been reconfigured to attempt to show how smaller hospitals of no more than 100 bedrooms (and some with no beds at all) can be used as a critical mass suitable for most specialities. Larger hospitals might eventually be replaced by networks of smaller hospitals that go hand in hand with responsive local services providing continuing care at home, day-care or, if need be, residential care[9]. This smaller hospital building-led cry for action is seen by LB as a medium-term initiative (it is anyone's guess as to how long medium-term might be!). This could be seen by some who wish to discourage the use of new buildings and infrastructure as a worst-case scenario because these are major contributors to carbon emissions but the whole purpose of this message is that "less means more," "small is beautiful", "something is better than nothing", "God rolls his own", "who gives a damn about apathy?" and "Let's do it".

If the NHS cannot make smaller hospitals work for its patients in their local community then our living longer lives will become much harder to endure – please believe

---

[9] Watch this space! The European Healthcare Design Congress meets in London on 9-11 June 2025. There has been a call for papers dealing with "Beyond the Hospital – form, function and the future healthcare system". This intends to uncover a new healthcare system for health and wellbeing. LB hopes this does not fall in line with the promotion of larger European super hospitals, even those that try to mimic Le Corbusier.

LB, he knows it and is doing just that (ask RG!) along with millions of others.

As of 31st October 2024 (following the budget announcements) the waiting list for surgical and medical procedures stood at 7.64 million – before Covid it was just over 4 million

Acknowledgements

See the first two *Dear Susan...* paperbacks listing some of the cast of hundreds (maybe even thousands!) with many thanks.

This list mentioned Stuart Robinson who is still with us but is now unable to remember his major contribution. Stuart produced operational policies based on government/NHS policy guidance for the second tranche of Nucleus Hospitals data packs. These operational policies have filtered down to inform the PLANS included in Chapter 2 of this third Dear Susan... paperback. Perhaps it is also now time for LB to stop remembering!

Special thanks to Dear Susan, Lord D and Dear Mungo, and anyone working on developing social/educational policies to actively support a notion that healthy living reduces a need for some surgical and medical interventions.

Appendix

PLAN X over page uses an existing hospital site to illustrate how a number of smaller hospitals might be placed together. This is less like a district general hospital and more like a science park. The trauma and elective care centres are positioned at the entry to the site for speedy access, the emergency care centre is located centrally for referrals from the community and the other small hospitals on site. Women and children are located further into the site in a less urgent environment and the chronic care centre in a more tranquil setting.

Smaller hospitals should ideally be located on their own sites to be where they are needed and to stand alone. The site shown in **PLAN X** was formerly a brown field site purchased by an NHS trust in 1990 to build the last nucleus hospital. This site plan is used here to illustrate how five smaller hospitals might be set out on this site to stand alone from each other but please look back to Chapters 1 and 6 to understand why large hospitals, even those using multiples of smaller hospitals are less relevant to a changing NHS.

APPENDIX

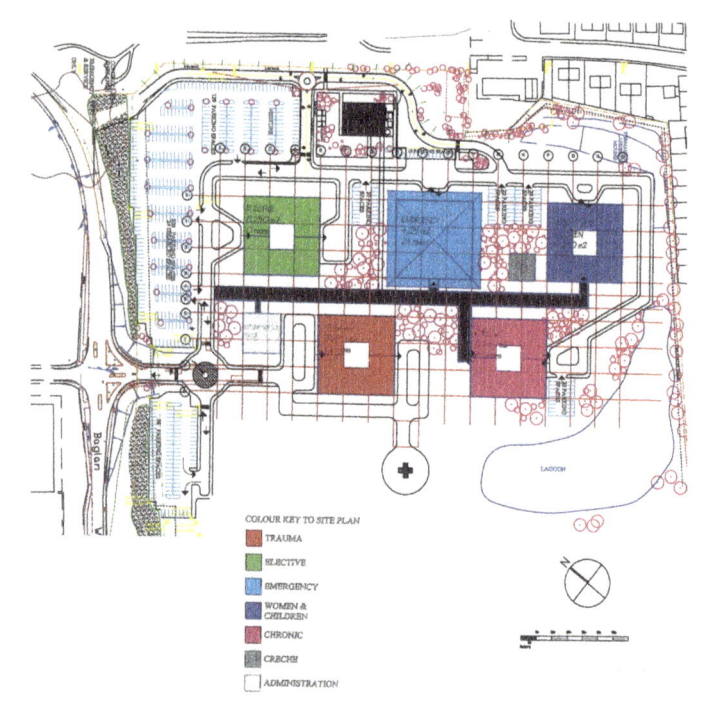

PLAN X

PLAN X. This shows how five smaller stand-alone hospitals of less than 10,000m² each might be grouped together on a single site – a worst-case scenario if expediency dictates that more than one should be built on an existing hospital site because it has always been there and is available!

A Chorus for all to sing!

Lyrics for a chorus are set down below[10]. These might be sung by those politicians and policy makers from the target audience set out in the Preface together with their advisers, support staff and hospital planners – every Monday morning:

"We're busy doin' nothin'

Workin' the whole day through

Tryin' to find lots of things not to do

The NHS is goin' nowhere

Isn't it just a crime

We'd like to have it sorted, but

We never do have the time

La la la la la la…"

---

[10] Borrowed with thanks with a slight rewording of the chorus – by Jimmy Van Heusen originally sung by Bing Crosby.

A final prompt!

This final prompt is a summary of the criterion set out in Chapter 1, which informed the plans in Chapter 2. It might usefully be remembered by readers as more and more people than are needed put their minds to sorting out the state of the NHS estate and its crumbling hospitals.

Smaller hospitals should:

Keep it simple
Keep patients in mind
Keep low – up to four-storey for patients
Keep below 10,000m² – smaller whenever possible
Keep control (stand-alone and secure)
Keep therapeutic and enterprising
Keep healing
And…
Keep replacing crumbling hospitals – quickly

The notice at the top of the noticeboard in Photo Five reads:

ED MISSION STATEMENT
WE DELIVER URGENT LIFE SAVING CARE IN A CHALLENGING ENVIRONMENT

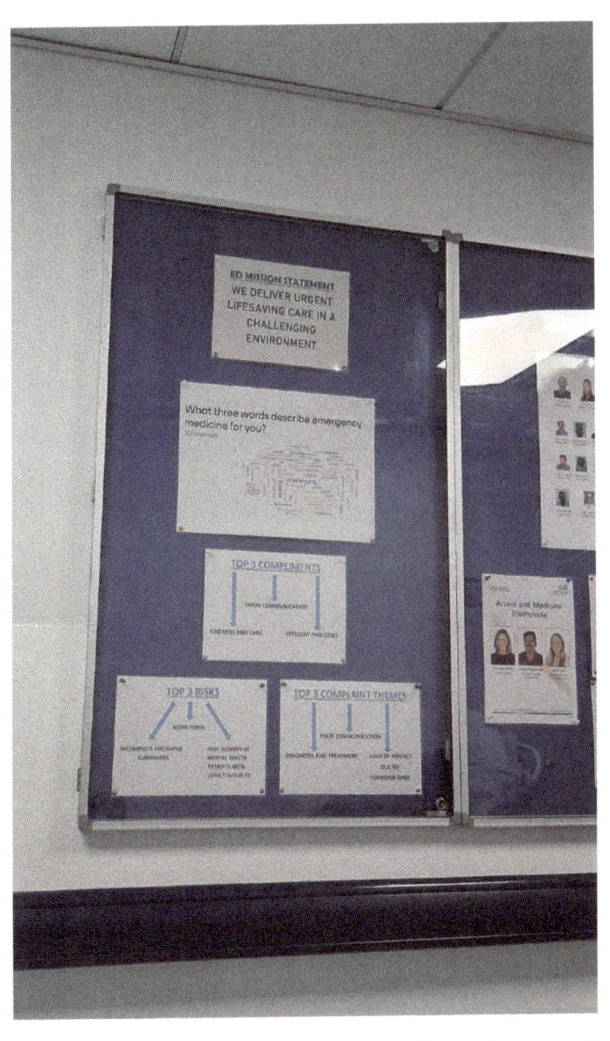

Photo Five. The above photograph of a patients notice board was taken by LB while receiving "corridor care" from a trolley at The Royal Surrey County Hospital, Guildford on 21st January 2025 (ED = Emergency Department)

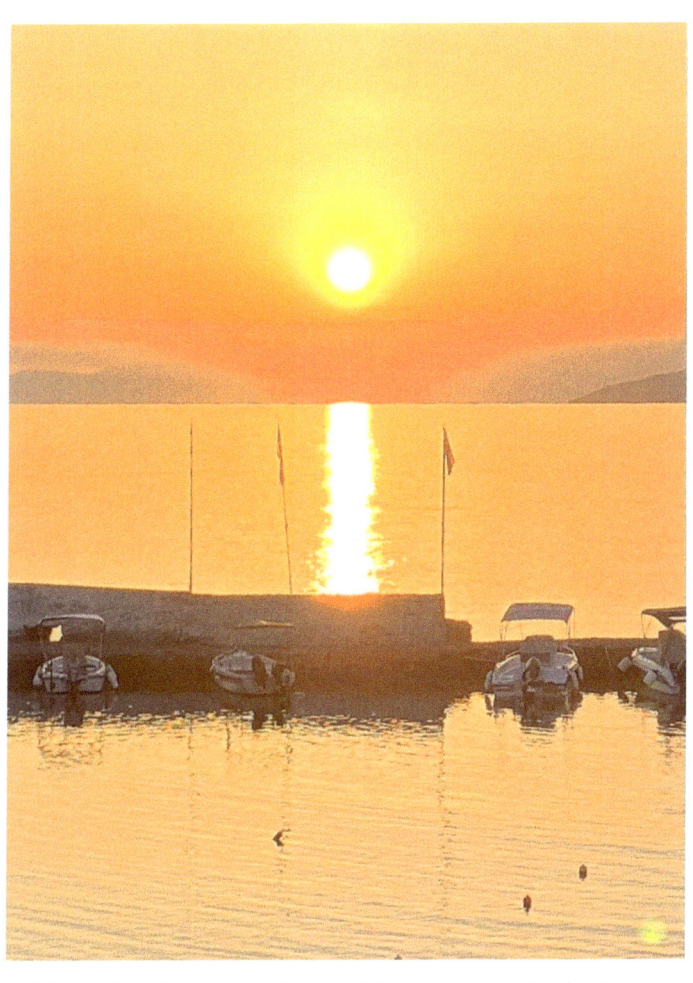

Photo Six. The going-down of the sun over the harbour wall – Greece. Or possibly the going-down of the sun on the NHS – or is there still hope?

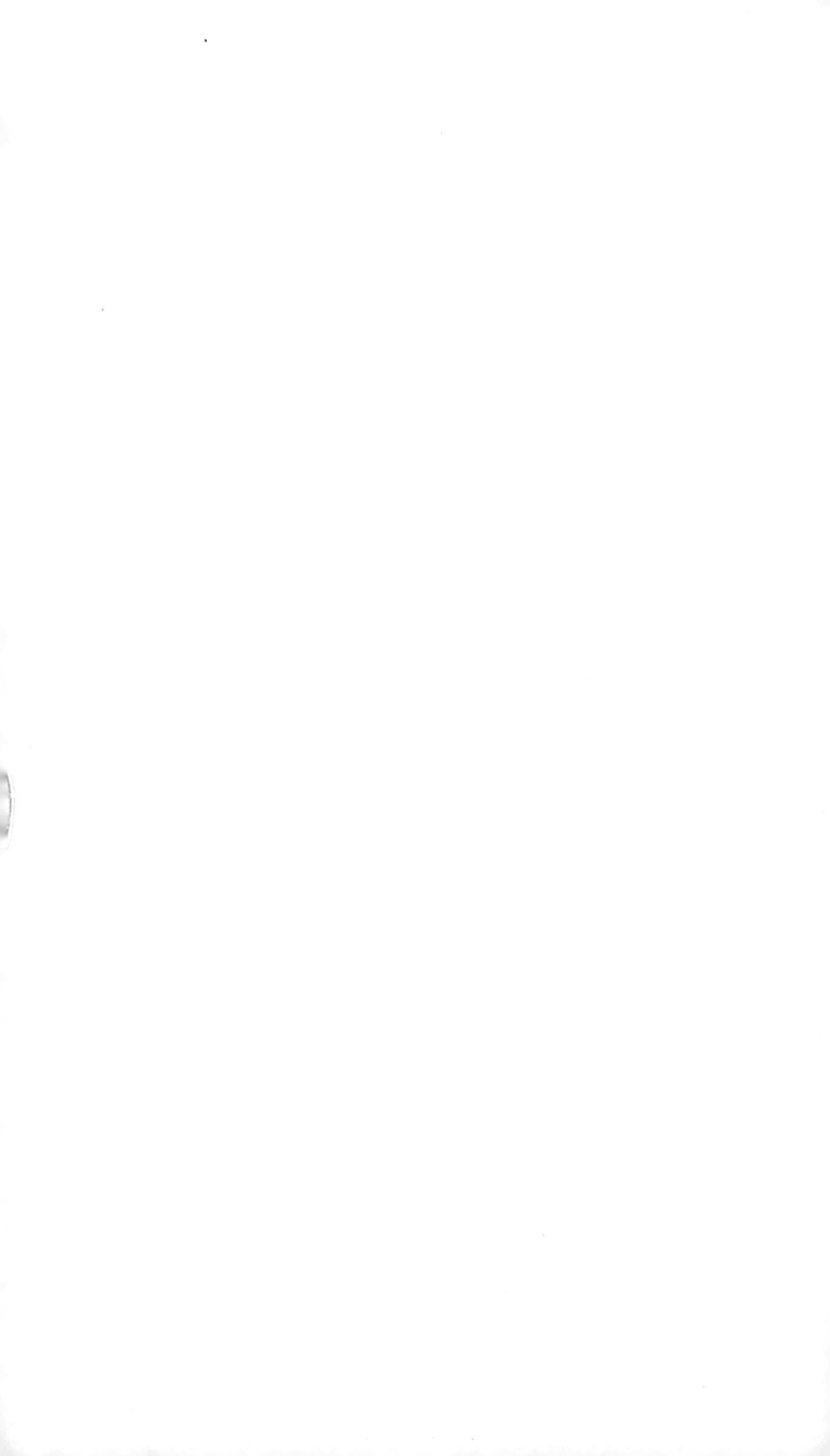